ADVICE
TO DOCTORS
& Other
Big People

From Kids

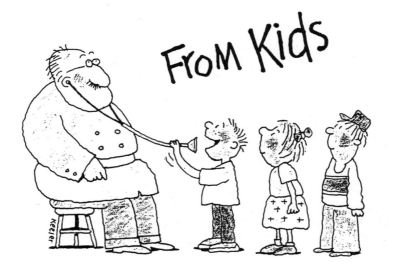

THE CENTER FOR ATTITUDINAL HEALING

Foreword by Dr. Gerald Jampolsky, M.D.

CELESTIALARTS

Berkeley, California

FIRST PRINTING, 1991

Library of Congress Cataloging in Publication Data

Advice to doctors & other big people from kids / The Center for Attitudinal Healing ; foreword by Gerald G. Jampolsky.
  p.   cm.
  ISBN 0-89087-618-5
  1. Terminally ill children—Psychology. 2. Children's drawings. 3. Center for Attitudinal Healing (Tiburon, Calif.). I. Center for Attitudinal Healing (Tiburon, Calif.).
II. Title: Advice to doctors and other big people from kids.
RJ249.A38   1990
610.69'6—dc20   90-38755
                                                                                       CIP

1	2	3	4	5	6	7	8	9	0	/	95	94	93	92	91

*Happy is the time when the great
listen to the small,
for in such a generation
the small shall listen to the great.*

—Talmud

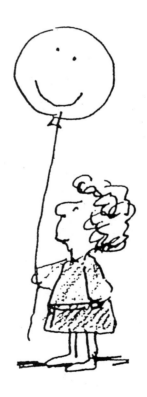

Contents

Introduction and Dedication

This book was written by children who have come to the Center for Attitudinal Healing in Tiburon, California, for support during their treatment for catastrophic illness. These children became both students and teachers to one another, as well to those of us big people lucky enough to be there to listen.

Many of these children have recovered and moved on with their lives; some are still in treatment, their futures uncertain; some have died.

We dedicate this book to those of our young teachers who have passed on, in love and thanks for the many lessons they so beautifully taught us while they were here in Earth School:

Ricky Alaniz

Valerie Fraser

Earl Garcia

Christina Marconi

Noah Wolfson

— ♥ —

Thanks!
From the Authors

Advice to Doctors and Other Big People ... From Kids is the result of a collaborative project that has been ongoing at the Center for Attitudinal Healing for several years. Many wonderful people have contributed their time and heartfelt energy to this book.

We especially wish to thank the members of our families who wrote from their own experience, contributing to Chapter 10, "What It's Like for the Family."

We wish to thank our editor, Dale Going, and also our associate editors, Kay Atwood, Jack Gaines, Diane Grinsell and Cynthia Sirkin. Their commitment, persistence, time and loving attention made this book possible.

Thanks to our designer, Louise Franklin; to cartoonist Jack Keeler, who did the cover illustration; and to the many children at the Center who contributed their drawings to this book.

Special thanks to Gerald Jampolsky, Phoebe Lauren, Kathy Harris, Cheryl Shohan, Lynn Scott, Carolyn Smith, Geri Brooks, Jody Paymer, Maggie Morgan, Annie Reardon and the many volunteers at the Center who have been a part of our groups and a part of our lives.

Most of all, thank you to our parents, our brothers and sisters, our doctors and nurses. Your love helps us heal.

— ♥ —

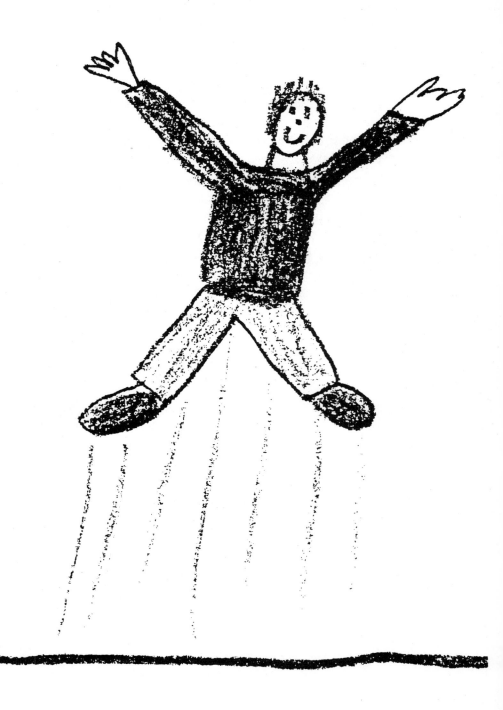

About the
Center for Attitudinal Healing

The Center for Attitudinal Healing was established in 1975 to supplement traditional health care by providing an environment in which both children and adults faced with life-threatening illness can actively participate in the process of attitudinal healing.

The concept of attitudinal healing is based on the belief that it is possible to choose peace rather than conflict and love rather than fear. We believe that love is the most important healing force in the world. Attitudinal healing is the process of letting go of painful, fearful attitudes. When we release fear, only love remains. At the Center, our definition of health is inner peace, and healing is the process of letting go of fear.

— ♥ —

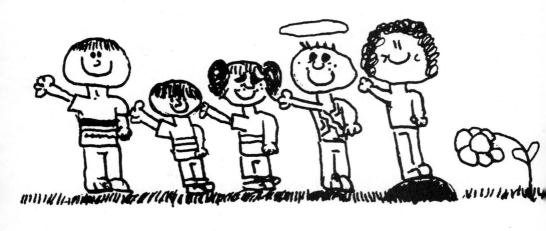

Foreword

There have been many books written by physicians, nurses and other members of the health professions about ways of working with children and their health problems.

This book is different. It is written by children.

Sometimes we adults become so busy with our day-to-day responsibilities that we don't take time out to listen with patience to what might be in the minds and hearts of the children we touch.

The purpose of this book is to give kids an opportunity to be heard, to offer their suggestions and to express some of their feelings to the doctors, nurses and other health care workers who are helping them with their healing. We hope, too, that it will help the adult reader to listen to the innocent child within.

We have all learned a great deal from the kids at the Center for Attitudinal Healing in Tiburon, California, where we have a strong belief that everyone is an equal teacher. We hope and trust that you find their thoughts of benefit to you.

Gerald G. Jampolsky, M.D.
Founder and Consultant
Center for Attitudinal Healing
Tiburon, California

— ♥ —

When little kids are real jumpy and nervous, they tend to need something to do. A fish tank where there are things moving around helps them calm down. It gets their minds off of getting shots and things like that.

—Kenny Estrada

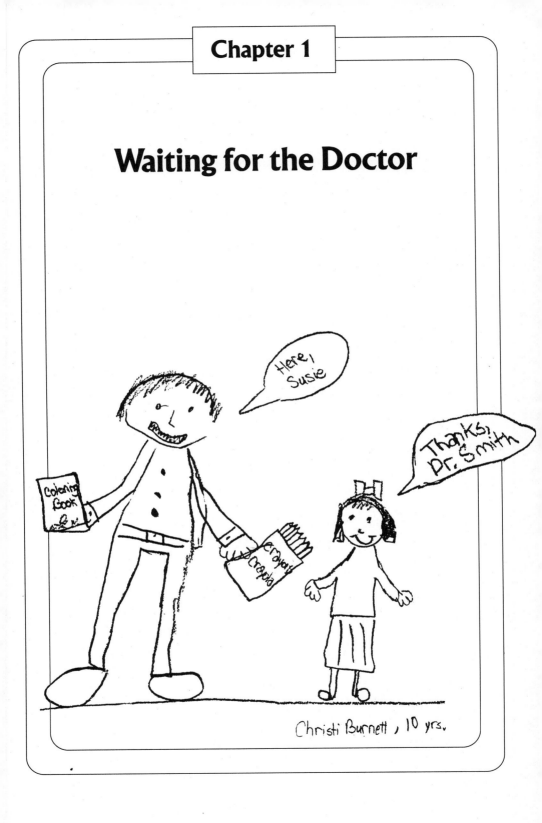

When you're waiting, you worry about what's gonna happen, how it's gonna happen, when it's gonna happen.

—*Kenny Estrada*

First you wait for the lab, then you wait to see if your count is down, then you wait for the doctor, then after the doctor sees you, you wait for the medicine, then you wait to get your next appointment, so there's a lot of waiting.

—*Valerie Fraser*

There's not really anything you can do to get rid of the anxiety that goes with waiting, because no matter what, you're still waiting.

—*Bobby Toops*

Once I had to wait four hours, and no one came out to tell me that I would have to wait longer. I feel trapped when I wait for a long time.

—*Josh Engholm*

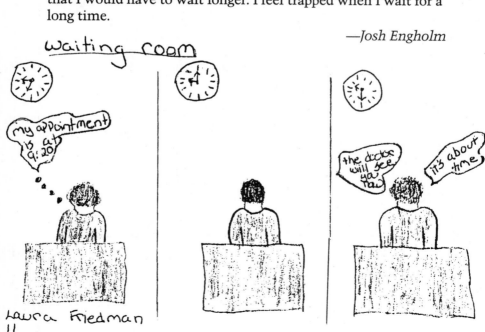

I'd put in lots of pillows.

—*Quincy Munch*

I'd put a rainbow on the wall.

—*Rhonda Bruntmeyer*

I'd get different magazines on different subjects, so there'd be something for everybody to read.

—*Bobby Toops*

If you have a playroom in a waiting room, you might run into the problem of the children getting excited and being noisy. It's not really relaxing to have young kids screaming in a waiting room, so there should be quiet stuff to do.

—*Maria Immel*

I would brighten the room up. I would have interesting books for people to read. I would have a pile of Lego blocks for kids to play with and I would put in comfortable booths in which people could sit or lie down.

—*Noah Wolfson*

The best thing about the waiting room at the clinic was Mark the Storyteller, who'd come and read books to us. The waiting room was yellow and blue. The windows opened up so you could get fresh air. There was a goldfish tank where I waited for radiation and there were Legos. But a lot of the toys were broken and a lot of the books were old and worn. It would be great to have new toys and books.

—*Zack Ward*

I really think that appointments should all be made with the thought that the patient is important, so they will see you on time. Otherwise, you feel like you don't matter, that the doctor's not thinking of you.

—*Eve Nadel*

It's boring. It's tense. The art looks terrible. The chairs are totally uncomfortable. The magazines have been read so many times that you can't make out the words. You think about the worst possible things you could and feel frustrated with the doctor for not being able to be there on time.

—*Noah Wolfson*

It's good if the nurses come out and talk with you while you're waiting.

—*Liam McCauley*

It's kind of fun when I'm waiting at the clinic. They weigh you each time you go. You have to wait maybe ten or fifteen minutes before you do that, so I play. After getting weighed the last time, I had to wait a really long time and my mom had time to read me three or four books.

—*Sarah Cox*

There aren't any good books at the doctor's office.

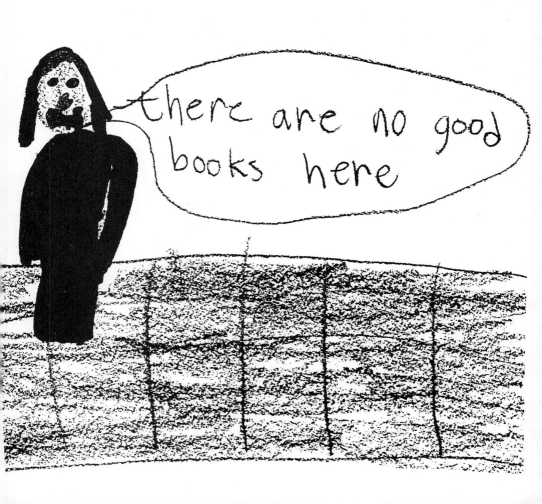

Doctors could let you know that no question is a dumb question, so you won't feel afraid to ask something.

—John Crandall

Chapter 2

Examinations

You're very nervous, even if it's not a big exam. You wonder if something is wrong, or if you'll have to have more shots and medicine. And you wonder why they don't always tell you the truth.

—*Noah Wolfson*

I really appreciate the doctors who let me know what they're doing as they're doing it. Sometimes they tell me what the tests they're giving me are for. It should be like that all the time. Sometimes they just do it and leave me there. Then it's scary, spooky.

—*Maria Immel*

When I have a blood test, I try to forget that the IV's in my arm. I try to think of something else, like my favorite place or being with my mom.

—*Marina Rozen*

I don't think the doctor is hurting me on purpose when he gives me a shot. He says it hurts him more. I forgive him. It helps if my parents are in the room. Breathing helps.

—*Zack Ward*

I like it when the doctors and nurses count "One, two, three," before they poke me. Or, they say, "Ready?"

—*Sarah Cox*

Doctors could make it easier by asking you if you're relaxed or whether it's your first time. They could give you information about everything you're going to go through, so you know exactly what will happen and how it will feel and to make sure that you're not afraid of something.

—*John Crandall*

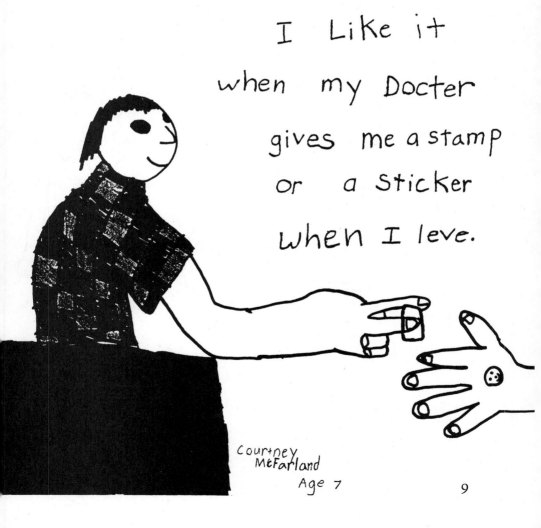

I Like it when my Docter gives me a stamp or a sticker when I leve.

Courtney McFarland
Age 7

What bothers me about x-ray machines is that they always make you wear heavy pads to protect you from radiation, then they desert you for several minutes while they go operate the machine. So I'm left there being crunched by this thing and not knowing what's going on, wondering if they're more interested in protecting themselves than me.

—*Maria Immel*

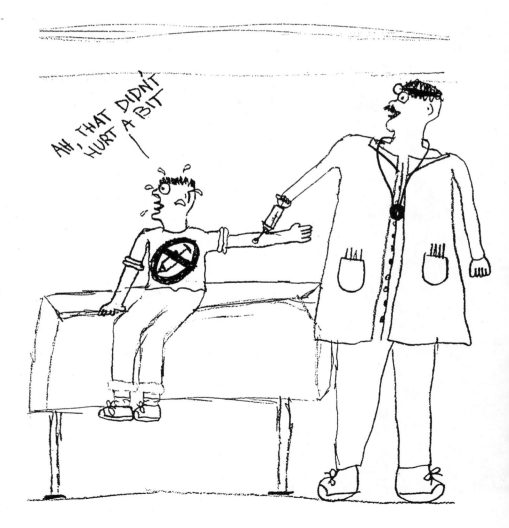

If something really hurts you physically or psychologically, you should be free to tell the doctor that you don't like it. The doctor should take that into consideration.

—*John Crandall*

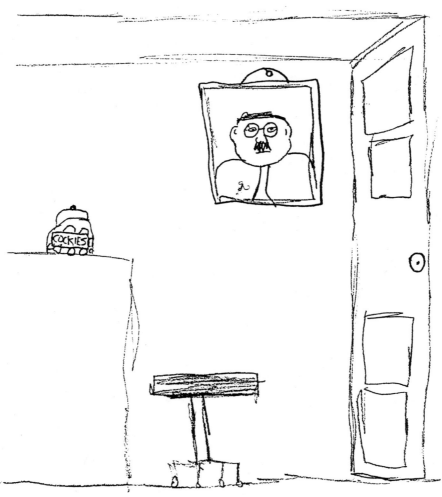

Drew Roulette

*I was pretty mad that the doctors
didn't tell me first that I had cancer.
They told my parents. It's the kid's
life and the kid should know about it.*

—Ricky Alaniz

Chapter 3

How Doctors Talk to Kids

My Doctor makes me laugh because hes funny.

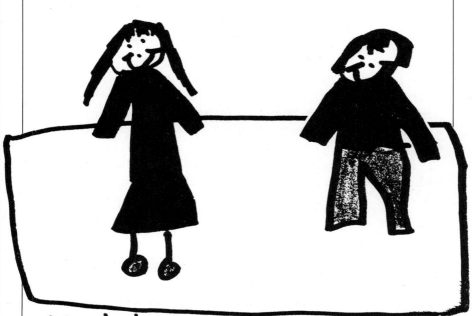

Nairi tashjian age 7

Some doctors use all the medical jargon with all these twenty-letter words. Others are nice enough to put it into the English language as most people know it.

—*Maria Immel*

It would help a lot if they wouldn't use such big words. It made it worse than it was. I thought I was doomed.

—*Margaret McDonald*

Most of the time, I trust my doctors. I trust them to take care of me. I don't trust them to tell me everything that's going on. I'd like my doctor to be honest. If a doctor reassures me, then I feel that it's worse than he's saying — that he's trying to hide something.

—*Maria Immel*

When I had my ileostomy, the doctor told my mom, but he only told me he was just going to take something out and it would be really simple. I thought it would only take an hour. Then I woke up 6 hours later and everything was all fuzzy around me and I tried to sit up. I heard this crinkling sound and I saw a bag was attached to me by my stomach. Then I was mad and I wished I'd been the doctor so I could do that to him.

—*Josh Engholm*

I hope what they're telling me is the truth.

—*Bobby Toops*

The doctor says — I don't know what he says. He uses big words.

—*Peter Elias*

14

I've been to different doctors and they've diagnosed me for completely wrong things, thinking that was definitely what I had. Doctors tend to want to think they know what's wrong, but a lot of times they really don't. I wish some of them would have said to me, "Really, I'm not sure what's going on with you, I can't help you."

—*Eve Nadel*

I had back surgery when I was fourteen. I was pretty angry at the way I was treated. They never conferred with me—I had no way of communicating even "yes" or "no" at that time, so they didn't understand that I was mentally functioning. My dad asked the doctor how long I would be in bed after the operation. "Nine months." I began to cry. The doctor responded quite uncompassionately. If I were a doctor, I would have shown the little guy some compassion and empathy.

—*Kelly Niles*

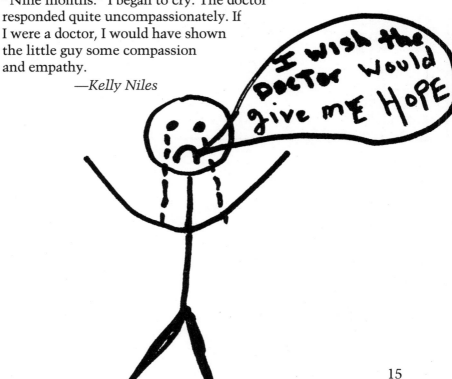

15

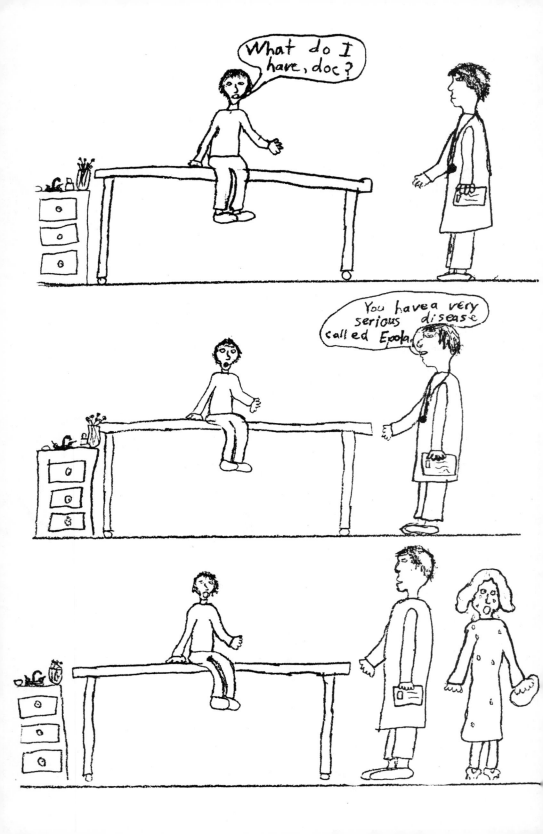

Doctors are usually very kind to me these days. A lot of it comes from my demanding that. I hate being patronized. I tell the doctors to talk to me directly and not to shout. Because I can't speak, people act as though I can't hear.

—*Kelly Niles*

I like the doctor to be pretty straightforward with me. I think with medications, it's really important to tell the patient what to expect, when to expect it, and tell them any complications or side effects they may have. When I first got diagnosed, they put me on a drug that made me really tired. I couldn't go to school because I'd just be falling asleep. I was angry that they didn't tell me this is a possible side effect which a lot of people have.

—*Eve Nadel*

I'd like my doctor to be more to the point. We had a conference but it wasn't clear enough for me. She said people don't want to hear just the straight facts. But I think if at the very beginning she had said that the chemotherapy was my only chance for a long-term recovery, I would have had a whole different attitude, a more positive attitude. I would have known this was it and given it the whole shot.

—*Valerie Fraser*

Sometimes I found out my test results from the doctors and sometimes from my parents. I'd like it to be that my doctors tell me with my parents there, a group meeting, so that everyone knows at the same time and you can ask any questions that need to be asked.

—*Maria Immel*

I felt like doctors were far away and there was a big separateness. I wished I could have talked to them more and known a little more about them.

—Josh Engholm

Chapter 4

How Kids
Talk to Doctors

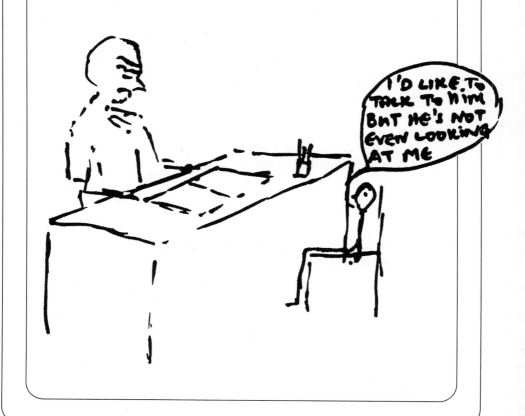

What I want to do about my illness is trust to get better, trust in the natural process to heal. I wonder if my doctor thinks that way.

—*Bobby Toops*

When your mind's in turmoil after finding something out, it's really hard to ask any questions or talk about it at all, so I don't think there's much a doctor can do to help explain things at first. They should try, but they shouldn't expect any response. Usually the kids hear; it just takes a while for them to really think about it.

—*Ricky Alaniz*

In the beginning I didn't understand what was happening — both because they didn't explain and because I didn't want to learn. After I overcame some of the fear I had about my sickness, I started to ask more questions, because I wanted to know more what was happening to me and what was going on inside of me with the drugs. I would have liked to know how other kids reacted to the drugs I was on, what I could expect and what I could do to make it easier.

—*Noah Wolfson*

When I'm feeling scared, I definitely cannot say that to the doctors. They don't seem reachable, somehow. It seems like they're just there to do a job. Once in a while, there's a friendly person, but usually I feel like they don't really care exactly how I feel.

—*Maria Immel*

20

I thought I was indestructible. I didn't think anything could stop me, and then all of a sudden, boom, I was really sick and I just felt really bad. It was about a week after the doctor told me that I had leukemia that it really hit me what I had. I didn't know what it was at that time. I started looking into it, started asking questions. But I just thought it was a big dream and that everything would be better. I think denial is the worst thing that I could have done to myself, because it put me into a deep depression. The doctors did their best to try to help me, but they really didn't help me get out of my depression. They just treated me for my cancer.

—*Earl Garcia*

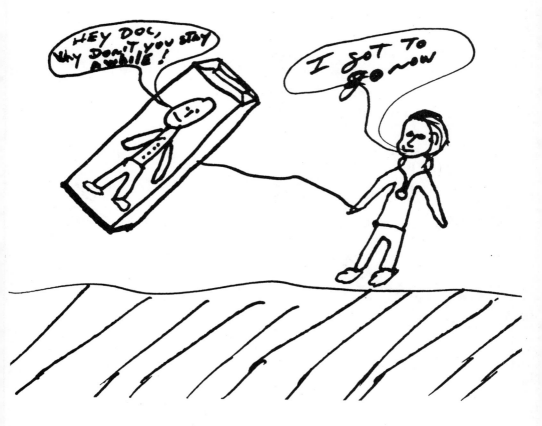

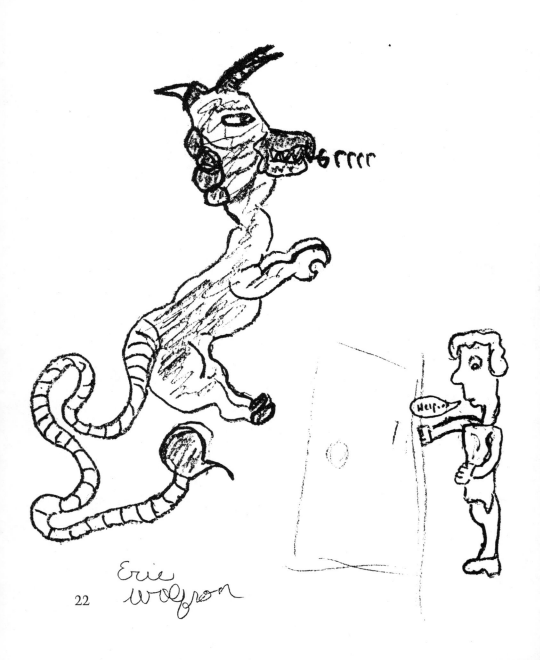

I don't always feel like I can talk to my doctor, because he's so business-like. I wish he would visit me.

—*Quincy Munch*

I wish I could talk to them more about teenage problems.

—*Ricky Alaniz*

I can talk well with my nurses, but they can't answer all my questions the way my specialist could. I didn't understand much of what he told me about the side effects—he told it too technically. I had to check out books to find out more about what I had.

—*Margaret McDonald*

I think I would have felt more comfortable if I knew something about the doctor and he knew something about me. A closer relationship would make it easier to talk or ask questions.

—*Maria Immel*

I think it's really important that a doctor listens to you as a human being instead of just treating you like an object that they're trying to cure or trying to help. To really listen to you, not necessarily to be able to solve everything but to listen and to understand how the patient's feeling.

—*Eve Nadel*

Don't treat us like babies.

—*Rhonda Bruntmeyer*

When I was in the hospital, they had toys for me to play with in the playroom. I had fun there. They had lots of videos that kids like to watch and we made things. There were arts and crafts, stuffed animals, games. I can't go to daycare or be with kids in other places because there are too many infections, but I can play with kids in the playroom at the hospital.

—Melissa Callen

Chapter 5

Being in the Hospital

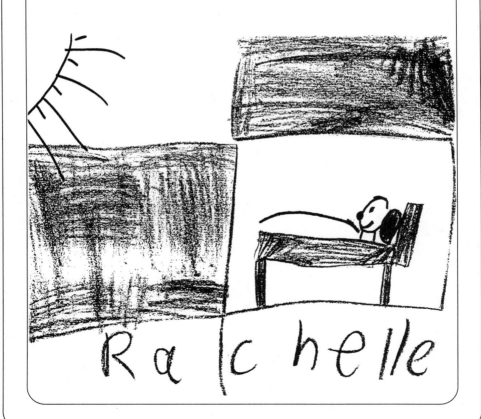

Rachelle

I was pretty dazed for quite a while after surgery, with pain medication. I do remember my doctor coming into my room with my family there and telling me that I had leukemia. I was still kind of out of it. Inside, I knew it was happening to me, but my body didn't want me to know that. I'd be in the hospital and I'd just say to myself, "I'm not here right now."

—*Earl Garcia*

When I went into surgery, I had been drugged and was only half there. But they seemed to care about me, because they showed me two caps for my hair, a blue cap and a flowered cap, and they asked me which one I wanted to wear. Somehow that just seemed like a nice thing to do.

—*Maria Immel*

They always either let my mom or my favorite nurse come in when I'm getting chemo. They hold my hand and tell jokes to cheer me up and that's good!

—*Margaret McDonald*

I'd make the operating room warmer, because it's cold down there.

—*Quincy Munch*

You get breakfast served in bed.

26

My mom had to sneak a radio in, because they were against hospital rules. I even had headphones, so I wouldn't bother the other patients — still I had to sneak to play it. Once, they said I'd only be in the hospital for a week. Then it was another, then another. It ended up being a whole month.

—*Rhonda Bruntmeyer*

You can't really sleep in the hospital because they wake you up every two hours to take your temperature.

—*Sarah Cox*

It felt okay if my parents left during the day, but I liked having them spend the night.

—*Melissa Callen*

When I had radiation, I almost fell asleep because you just lie there and you can't move at all. Everybody goes out of the room and it's real quiet and sometimes you hear some beeps. If you relax, it isn't scary.

—*Sarah Cox*

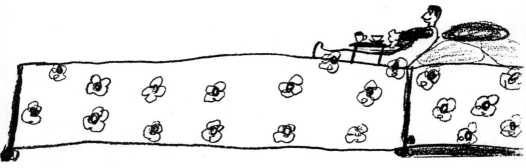

Naveen Baral

My doctor always asked if I wanted to have certain things done. She would say, "Do you feel okay about this?" She made me feel like I was really a part of my health, I was part of the team trying to get me better.

—*Eve Nadel*

Treatment is very hard and rigorous. You sometimes feel like you don't want to live anymore. I was really delirious. I changed moods every five minutes. I couldn't concentrate on anything, not even reading. I didn't know what I wanted out of life or why I wanted it. It was really hard for my parents and brother. I had horrible temper tantrums and said things I didn't mean.

—*Noah Wolfson*

I decided to stop chemotherapy because I just couldn't handle it anymore. My mom pretty much let me do what I felt was appropriate, though she helped me make the decision. We read books all weekend. When I finally told my doctor what I wanted, she told me the chemo is the only thing she knows that's going to do anything to help; that other treatments would only last another couple of months. So I decided not to quit. I think, since I've gone back, I've done better. I haven't felt sick at all. So it seems to have made a difference that I was given some voice.

—*Valerie Fraser*

The scariest part of it all is getting nauseous, because you feel like you're really losing it. It's scarier than all the shots and all the heavy machinery buzzing around you.

—*John Crandall*

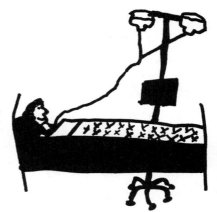

If you're a brain tumor patient, you're gonna lose your hair. It's very helpful if whoever is to shave you is able to do it with a nice manner. The lady who shaved my head made me so comfortable. She said, "Okay, how do you want it?" And I said, "Well, I've got to remove it all." She said, "No, it's your hair, you grew it, you get to choose how you lose it." "You mean, if I said, 'Give me a Mohawk,' you'd give me a Mohawk?" "That's right." So, she gave me a Mohawk. I was watching this in the mirror and then I said, "Far out! Now shave off the Mohawk and leave it on the sides," so I looked like who knows what. Then I just put down the mirror and said, "Okay, now shave it all off." I couldn't watch her shave it all off and I never saw myself totally bald. When I got out of surgery I was all bandaged, I looked like a cotton swab. By the time they took the bandages off, I had black fuzz and it grew back thicker. By the time I went to my junior prom, I had a half-inch of hair all around.

—*Justin Gregoire*

It was reassuring to know that people were there all the time watching my monitors. I trusted them to take care of me.

—*John Crandall*

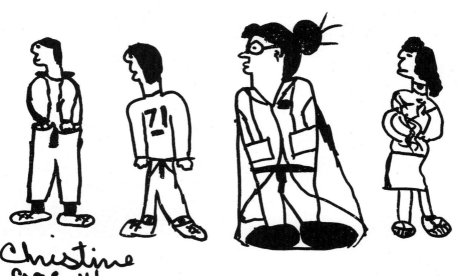

Christine
age 14

…what I have to say, to the patient and the doctor, is that you can accomplish anything as long as you try your best. Don't ever give up, no matter what.

—Andrew Watt

Chapter 6

Going Through Treatment

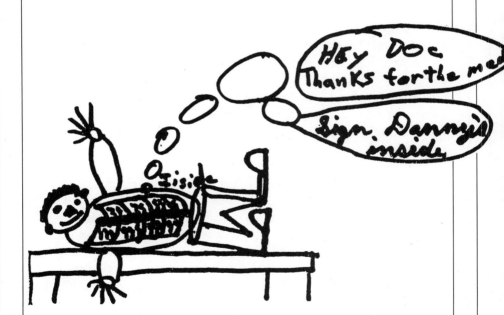

Andrew Watt was a member of the Children's Group at the Center during the last stages of treatment for a brain tumor that was discovered during a 14-hour surgical procedure. Since his recovery he has moved with his family to Ohio, where he is a junior high student. He shared the story of his treatment with us before he left.

— ♥ —

I was diagnosed with a brain tumor about three or four years ago, when I was eight or nine. I've been in the hospital lots of times. Once, near the end of my treatment, I stayed in the hospital for about six months.

When I first found out I had a brain tumor, it was kind of scary and I kind of didn't know what to think about it, being about eight or nine, you know how that is. I can't quite remember, but I think the doctor told my parents and my parents told me. About three weeks later, I had an operation.

One thing that helped me was to say, "I'm going to go through it. I'm not going to like it, but I'm going to go for it."

Another thing that helped was the fact that before the operation, until midnight, you get to stuff your face! My mom brought me a burger, some chips, a big gigantic soda, some candy!

Speaking of food, if you're a kid who is going through treatment and has to wait in waiting rooms, be sure to take a snack as well as something good to read. And — this is sort of advice for the doctors — put in a snack area, with free coffee or juice or cocoa, to keep us occupied. It would be great to have video games or TV in the waiting room.

When I was in the hospital, I think the nurses treated me pretty fairly. They did tell me, when they were going to stick the needle in, that it would just hurt a little bit, and that I would just be in a little pain, so that was okay. The first time I had an IV, my parents were there with me, but the second time, they weren't. I was with some nurses, and I could really see how cute and nice they were. That helped!

Sometimes when they gave me shots I'd tell them, "Watch out, because I'll get mad if you mess up." And they'd say, "Okay." Although, one time, about the second or third operation, when they were trying to stick the IV in, they didn't get it in a bunch of times. They had to give me the numbing needle again and they had to stick me a couple more times with the IV.

And when they put the gas mask on me to put me to sleep, I didn't know what to think. If it weren't for all those other nurses holding my arms down, I would have punched that guy, probably, because I had about had it. They said it would only take one time and here it took two or three times. That kind of made me mad. Their saying it would only take one time made me lack faith, gave me less confidence in them.

The thing that I really hated was the catheter. I remember the last time I had it, it took three nurses to hold me down when they took it out. I had been asleep when they put it in. I was awake when they took it out. They didn't explain anything, they just rushed in — at least that's the way it felt to me — and said they were going to take my catheter out. At first I was excited, but then when they did it, I felt like, "Whoa, I'm glad that's over with." It hurt! Of course it hurt! The way that they keep it in is by filling it with air. They released it and all this air went out and it made my stomach hurt. They didn't tell me to expect the air. They just said they were going to take it out, no problem, it would just take two minutes. It would have helped if they had said what to expect.

What I really liked about the nurses is that when I flirted with them, they talked back, they'd be kind of hard to get, and that kept me going. And when I first starting getting up, I was kind of dizzy. Most of the nurses would say, "Hi, Andy! You're up out of bed! Wow, you're slowly but surely recovering!" That encouraged me.

I pretty much liked all my doctors. Every day I'd get up and do something like go visit doctors. I was getting pretty popular in the hospital. I knew my way around. From the fifth floor down, I knew everybody there. Every day I would meet a new person. One thing I liked, I would go down to the cafeteria to eat with a nurse or a doctor. One of my favorite doctors — she was a really neat doctor — would always take me down to the "chow hall" as they call it, to get a burger. It was better than the food upstairs. I think she did this because she cared about me a lot. That made me feel good. Some of my doctors were like that, took that kind of time with me.

The most important thing my doctors did was not give up on me. They didn't say things like, "Oh well, the odds are too big, I'm not taking that risk." They really pulled for me. When the doctors here in San Francisco located the cancer, they went to a very delicate part of the brain, the pineal gland, actually, and they got a little piece of tissue to see what kind of tumor it was, to see what kind of treatment I needed. Back then, I had a tube from my first operation in Hawaii. The tube was for the water to escape from the pineal gland, so I wouldn't have a bloated head. I was kind of scared about that. They said if I had not gone to a doctor, in eight months I would have been either severely paralyzed for life or dead. But I got there in time and they were willing to risk doing that very delicate operation. I was really grateful to them for that.

My doctor in San Francisco was one of the best neuro-surgeons. He's very famous. You could go see him, you could go ask, "Do you know where Dr. B. is?" and they'd say, "Oh, sure! He's over there!" My doctor in Hawaii had been saying

34

things like, "Okay, we'll just give you this," without even knowing what I had. He basically told my dad there's nothing much they could do. My dad didn't want to take that risk, so he arranged for us to go to San Francisco for a second opinion. Two or three days before we left, my dad and my mom talked to the doctor and explained what we were gonna do. That doctor was pretty mad because he felt kind of insulted and kind of jealous. He doesn't know that I've recovered. I don't think he wants to be bothered.

But maybe he'll read this book. Maybe he would learn from that, because what I have to say, to the patient and the doctor, is that you can accomplish anything as long as you try your best. Don't ever give up, no matter what.

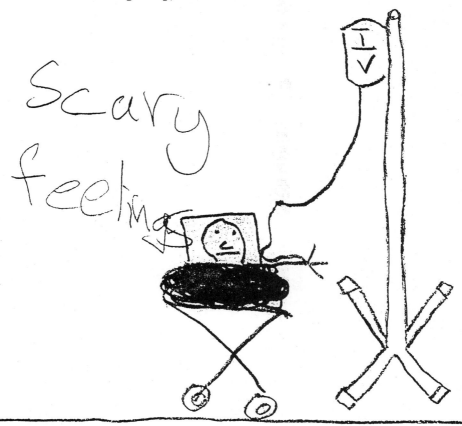

The best part about the doctor is when he gives me bubble gum. The worst part is when he's in the room with me and my mom and he only talks to my mom. I've told him I don't like that, but he doesn't listen.

—Marina Rozen

Chapter 7

Doctors

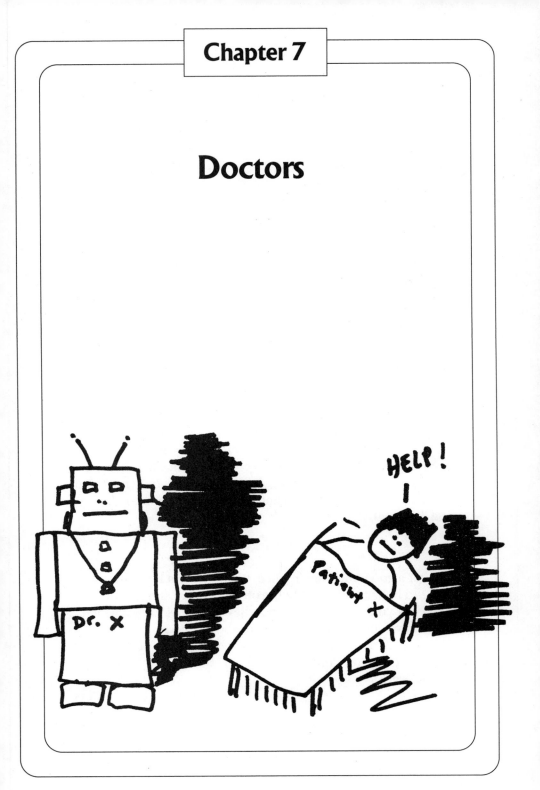

A doctor is a big thing that's not very reachable. Kind of solid, like a block of cement. You can't talk to it and it doesn't talk to you.

—*Maria Immel*

They let you know who's boss — they don't mess around. They're always so busy.

—*Quincy Munch*

I feel small and dumb around doctors, because I don't know what they're talking about all the time. And scared when they are possessed with the power of the needle.

—*Noah Wolfson*

When I met my doctor, I was really taken aback by him. I looked at him and I thought, "Jeez, this guy's a nerd!" He looked like your typical nerd with crew cut, big glasses, and I was thinking, "This guy's not going to be able to help me." But I opened up, I listened to him and he does know what he's doing, he's really good.

—*Justin Gregoire*

If you get a *good* one, they're nice, warm, have a fair amount of time to be with you and help you with every step to your recovery. If you get a *famous* one, they're always busy, rushed, usually have stand-ins, but also care about you. If you get a *bad* one, they don't know what they're doing, don't care, all they want is money, and you wonder if they forged their medical degree.

—*Noah Wolfson*

You don't always understand that doctors are just doing their job when they hurt you.

—*Bobby Toops*

My doctor calls me names and tickles me. I tickle him back. He calls me "Honey Bunny," "Pumpkin Pie," "Sweet Cakes." He's great because he tells me funny stories.

—*Melissa Callen*

When I was in the hospital, all the doctors teased me, and I hate being teased when I'm sick. Maybe I'm feeling sorry for myself, I don't know exactly, but I'm not in the mood to hear a stupid joke and laugh at it or be teased.

—*Maria Immel*

I like that my doctor's conscientious and thorough; even if someone tells her she's crazy, she'll still follow through and make sure everything's fine.

—*Valerie Fraser*

If I were a doctor, I'd take a lot of vacations so I'd be able to deal with all the death and stuff. I'd try to make it so people wouldn't worry too much. I'd try to reassure them when I could but I wouldn't lie to them. I'd make sure they know that there is a possibility that they'll be okay.

—*Quincy Munch*

Kids would like to know that doctors care.

—*Bobby Toops*

You've got to be able to be friends with your nurses. Friendly nurses is the key. If you don't have a friendly nurse, how can you relate to anyone there? Basically, in the hospital, they're your friends. Because when visiting hours are over, who's there?

—Justin Gregoire

Chapter 8

Nurses

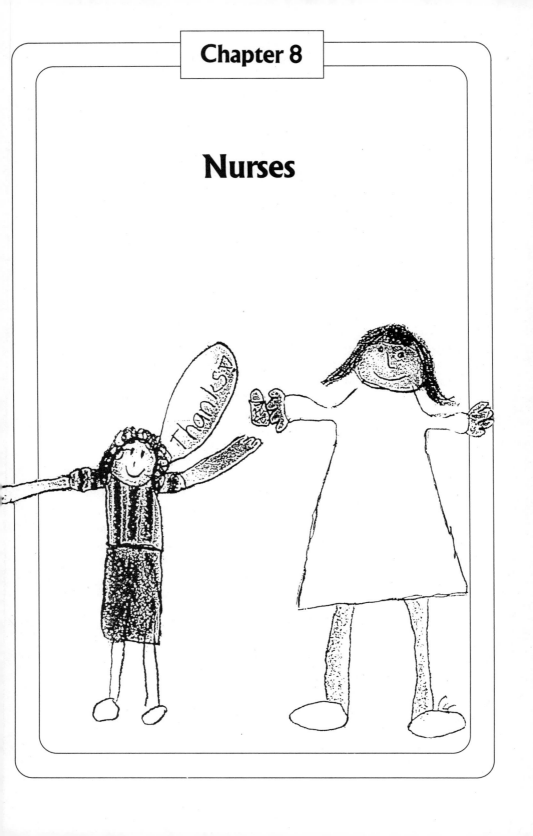

A nurse should take a little of the place of the parent. If shots were especially scary, I usually needed someone to hold my hand, and a nurse would be there. They should be able to talk to you and calm you down, even if their job is just to hold you down.

—*Kenny Estrada*

Most nurses are friendly and will talk to you when you need someone to talk to, like when you're feeling really bad because you've just found out you have to stay in the hospital an extra week, or when your parents aren't around. But also there are some nurses who just tell you what to do and you don't get any choice. Like, if you want something to drink and they're out of that, some nurses will order down to the cafeteria for more, but some will just say you have to have something else.

—*Bobby Toops*

When I think of nurses, I think of someone who should take as much time as they can to make you feel really at home when you're in the hospital, because you get really homesick. With some of them I felt like we were friends. It's more than just being there when you're needed. It's joking around, playing games. I know nurses have a lot of paperwork to do, but the good nurses put that aside and come spend time with you.

—*Margaret McDonald*

I think nurses work too long and people expect too much of them. They should be given the opportunity to leave if they've got a headache or aren't feeling well. If they were, I think you could save a lot of patients from getting a nurse's bad mood.

—*Maria Immel*

One of the nurses taught me how to take shots. She said, "You keep tensing up, that's why it hurts so much. What you need to do is just relax. The best way to relax is to watch as I do it." I put out my arm and she said, "Okay, here's the needle. You know me, I'm not going to hurt you. I'm going to put the needle in your vein and inject the fluid and I'm going to pull it out." I didn't even wince. I said, "It didn't hurt!" She said, "That's right. What makes it hurt is your brain. You're saying to yourself, 'I'm getting a shot and it's gonna hurt.' You need to relax." That's what she said, "Just relax. Put your hands at your side. Relax. Give me your hand." No problem.

—*Justin Gregoire*

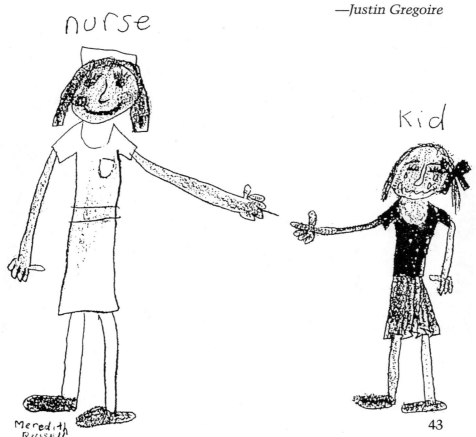

nurse

Kid

Meredith
Russell

Nurses should tell good jokes, give kids something to do when they have to wait a long time and take them for walks. I only got to go on one walk the whole time I was in the hospital.

—*Josh Engholm*

My Snoopy's tail was falling off and the nurse came in and sewed him up. She gave me little stickers that said "I had my shot" and she gave my Snoopy a sticker too, playing along that he was really real.

—*Maria Immel*

I remember one night I couldn't sleep, so I rang the bell. The nurse came in and I said, "Is it possible for me to get a sleeping pill? I can't sleep." She said, "Well, it's too late to give you a sleeping pill, but what I can do is give you a back massage."

—*Justin Gregoire*

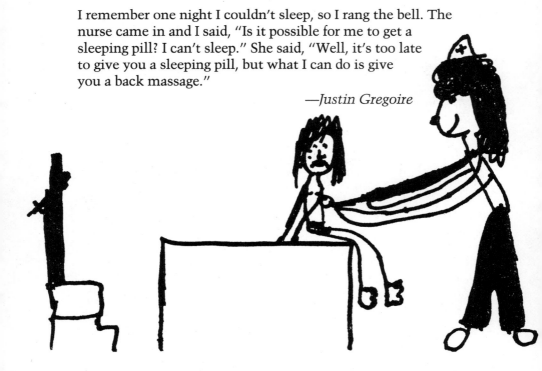

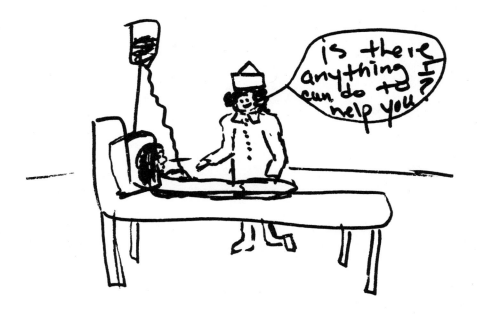

One night I was finally comfortable with myself, relaxing in my bed. A nurse came in and started taking my temperature and my blood pressure and all that stuff. It was like, "This is my job and let's get it over with." The night shifts, especially, want to get everything done so they can go relax. She turned on a blinding light above me, right in my eyes. I was awakened so suddenly. It really didn't feel good.

—*Earl Garcia*

One nurse, when I had to get a shot, called another nurse to hold my leg down. I'm always really good about being still and I didn't like it. I started crying because I always get really nervous before shots and I was yelling that I didn't want her, so she went away. It was better after that. At least they listened to me.

—*Sarah Cox*

If I had discovered cancer at twenty-one rather than at eleven, I would have asked a lot more questions than I did. Doctors ought to listen to kids and give them information — they just kind of bypass them.

—Nancy Peugh

Chapter 9

Looking Back

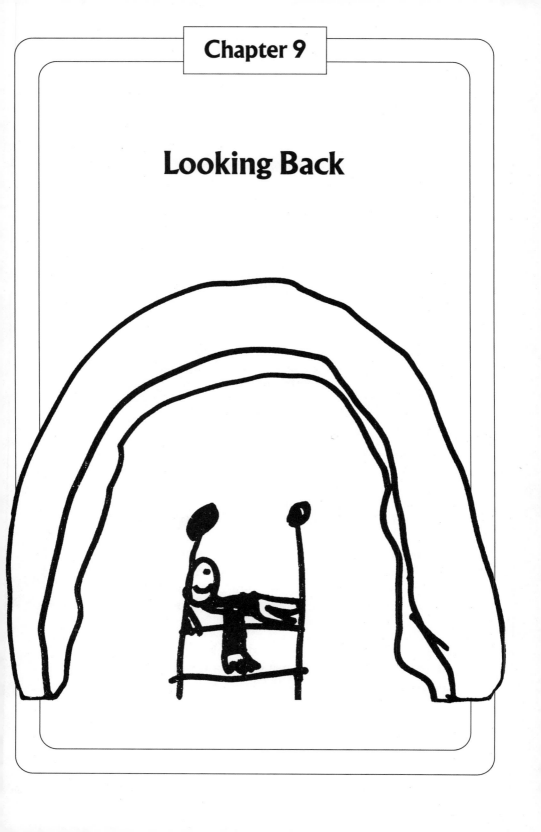

*Like most good friends, Nancy Peugh and Linda Stover
have a history of shared experiences, which they discovered
as members of the Young Adults Group at the Center for
Attitudinal Healing. Nancy was one of the children who
started the Center in 1975; Linda became involved with the
Center in 1981. They are close in age and have both recovered
from cancer, although with a ten year difference in their age at
diagnosis. From their unique and shared perspectives, Linda
and Nancy speak for the child that is within each of us,
regardless of age or experience.*

— ♥ —

Nancy — I was eleven when I had my first bout with cancer. We
were going away on a ski trip. My parents talked to the doctor and
then told me, "We're not going skiing. You're going into the
hospital." I fought it right out. I said, "No, I won't!" Accept that!
In the afternoon you're going skiing, and the next morning you
are in the hospital!

I kept saying I wasn't going to stay. I didn't carry anything in,
but my parents had my suitcase, so I thought *they* were staying.
A doctor came in and said, "Okay, let's check you out," looking
directly at me. He didn't know who I was. How did he know what
was happening to me? He told me I had something growing inside
that had to be taken out. I didn't know until several days later
that I had cancer of the kidney. I didn't know what cancer was.

They removed the kidney and I went through two years of
chemo and radiation. You know, going through extensive surgery
or chemo or radiation doesn't prove whether you're going to live
or die.

Linda — That's right. I always used to ask my doctor for a
guarantee. And he'd say, "I wish I could give you one."

I was diagnosed with non-Hodgkins lymphoma a week before
my twenty-first birthday. The doctors told my parents they never

expected me to see twenty-two. I'm glad I wasn't told that. I had a strong will to live and I was going to fight. Later, when I heard about it, I said, "Don't ever put a time limit on my life." Yet, they were honest with me about what I was going to go through. I knew that the chances weren't good. One day my doctor said, "You're a fighter and I know you can do it." He had put a lot of faith in me and in our working together.

I had gone to the doctor because I was having problems breathing. I had no idea I had cancer. As he was doing the examination he said to me, "Honey, there's a possibility that you have cancer. We need to put you in the hospital for a biopsy." I had been around cancer before — my grandfather died of it. I knew what a biopsy was. His attitude and his tone really made a difference. He realized my confusion and my fear and he was very gentle with me.

My doctor and I had a wonderful relationship, except that in the beginning of my treatment he had a hard time talking to me. I'd ask him a question and he'd either look at the wall or he'd look at my parents. He was used to dealing with the elderly and I was the youngest patient he had. I knew it was hard for him to talk to me because of my age, but I'd say, "I need you to talk to me, I need to know what's going on."

Nancy — I think it's very important to be open and honest with a child. Just because the doctor's sixty years old and he's talking to a child should make no difference. The child is no less human than the doctor. The doctor should talk to him so that he will understand and feel okay and then go ahead with whatever the treatment is.

Linda — A few months after I was diagnosed, I read that the treatment for non-Hodgkins lymphoma could effect my ability to have children. I called my doctor, and he said, "I told you that."

And I said, "No, you didn't." We talked about it and finally I realized that he *had* told me — the same day that I was diagnosed. When you hear you have cancer, you've got to absorb that. And then later — let the rest sink in.

Nancy — If I had discovered cancer at twenty-one rather than at eleven, I would have asked a lot more questions than I did. Doctors ought to listen to kids and give them information — they just kind of bypass them.

Linda — I've had some bad experiences with doctors, too. The radiation treatment burned my throat so badly that I couldn't swallow. I was brought into emergency to see my doctor and a throat specialist. The specialist held my tongue and talked to my doctor for five minutes as though I wasn't even there. Finally, I bit him. He jumped back and I said, "I'm a human being, please treat me like one!" He was angry and told my doctor that he'd never work with me again. But you know, sometimes I think they need a little compassion. They need to remember that.

   Once, near the end of treatment, when my veins were starting to collapse, I had to have an IV for a CAT scan. The oncology nurse offered to put the needle in because she'd worked with me, she knew my veins. I told this to the doctor but he said, "She's hard to get hold of, let me try." He tried five times. He kept insisting that he could do it. I finally got up and said, "I'm leaving unless you get her." She came and put it in the first time. He was irritated because I had faith in the nurse and I didn't have faith in him.

Nancy — At the hospital, I'd be told, "No more shots, you're finished for the day." Then five minutes later someone else would come in and start giving me more shots. I'd say, "Wait a minute, they told me I was finished for the day." "Well, I'm sorry, but this is what they need." Doctors, adults, just don't listen to an eleven year old child. They're going to pacify you, say, "Oh, don't worry about it, it's okay."

Linda — Obviously they went into that profession because they really cared, but sometimes they get so involved in their work that they don't realize what it's like for the patient.

One time when I was extremely sick, I had been sent to the radiology department for emergency work. I was on a bed because I was too weak to walk. I got left in the hall for an hour and a half. I sat there and yelled for someone, but no one responded.

The next time they left me in the hall, I was in a wheelchair and had a little more strength. I waited about ten minutes and decided not to wait any longer. I walked back to my room and left my wheelchair sitting there. The hospital was in an uproar because I took it upon myself to go back to my room. They don't realize that when you're really sick, to sit and wait for somebody to take you back to your room is just awful!

Nancy — It's the waiting that kids hate. It might be an hour. But to a kid, even ten or fifteen minutes is a *long* time!

Linda — A doctor and a patient are involved in a healing process and you need trust in that type of relationship. Let's say you like a doctor and the doctor says, "I'll be back in a few minutes," and keeps you waiting an hour. You're just not going to believe that doctor anymore.

Nancy — One time, this doctor came in to give me a shot. After he'd put on the tourniquet and I'd pumped my hand so the veins would come up, he was called away on an emergency phone call. He walked out of the room without taking the tourniquet apart. My arm was turning color and the nurse wouldn't unstrap my arm. She just sat there. Finally she called the doctor back and said, "Doctor, you forgot something."

Linda — I needed to have trust in my doctor. I felt that, regardless of what happened, I needed to be honest with him and I needed him to be the same with me. He was great about being there for me. He'd rearrange his whole schedule so he could personally give me my chemo. One time, he was going away for the weekend and while he was away I had to go into emergency and he showed up. I was very lucky. I knew he cared. He is just a fantastic man, very sympathetic.

When I first started chemo, I had to be hospitalized for four days each time and my doctor would come in the room and give me the chemo. At first, we wouldn't talk much. As treatment went on, we talked a lot more and it was more comfortable. And while I hated chemo, just knowing that we had that friendly rapport made it so much easier to take.

Nancy — When you're young, you see these big doctors in white coats and they're mountains compared to you down here. You don't know what to ask and you're so scared of them. But after a few days, I got used to my doctor. He came in and we played and talked and it wasn't all that bad.

Linda — I think it is really important to see the human side of the doctor. My tumors had not been responding to treatment. One day my radiologist came running in. He was jumping up and down. All of a sudden he kind of composed himself and said, "By the look of these records, your tumor is just starting to shrink!" Just by that, I could see a new side of the man and that he cared for me. It was good to see how human he was.

My oncologist always kept me posted on what was happening. I could feel his excitement. It was really important to me. I knew my doctors really cared about me. I wasn't just a case to them and that made a difference.

Nancy — I had a good rapport with my pediatrician and nurses, too. They would let me see my x-rays and look under the microscope to count my own white and red blood cells. It made it like a game I could play and understand. These little games gave me a part in my healing.

Linda — I think, too, that it's vital to realize how important family and friends can be. There was a sign on my hospital room door that said I was allowed no more than two visitors at a time, for no more than fifteen minutes. One time when I had five friends in my room, a nurse I'd nicknamed Sergeant, because she looked so strict and stern, walked in. She looked at us, counted, "One, two, three, four, five," said, "I only see two," and walked out.

Nancy — In my family, I was the most protected child. My brothers and sisters thought I was spoiled because I had cancer and was getting all the attention. They thought I was special and I felt the complete opposite. In the beginning, they didn't want to have anything to do with it. I didn't want them there either at first — I wanted my parents. But after awhile, they came when they realized what was going on and they wanted to help. I think siblings should be kept informed, not treated like they're in the way. The parents might want to hold back certain things that might scare the other siblings, but at least tell as much as they can.

Linda — I have a younger sister who was twelve when I was diagnosed. She really needed attention and I was getting all of it. My parents were open with her about what I was going through and she dealt with it really well. She joined a family support group at our hospital. My older sister has always been very protective of me, so she had a really hard time dealing with my illness. She sat by my hospital bed for a good four days and didn't say a word. I was trying to cheer *her* up.

I had a bad experience with a priest who came in and tried to convince me that I had to accept my death, because to him cancer was synonymous with death. He went to the point of giving me Last Rites. I couldn't get him out of the room. I kept telling him, "I'm not going to die," and he'd say, "You're denying it." When the nurses finally got him out, he cornered my sister and told her that she had to accept my death. My sister flipped out, thinking that my parents hadn't been honest with her. She went to my social worker. It made her finally open up, but it could have been really damaging.

In the beginning, I really believed I was going to live and that my faith was all I had. Later, when I was on my third chemo, down to a hundred pounds and puking my brains out, I told my mother, "I can't live the remainder of my life like this." My mother said, "The choice is yours." And that's when I chose to live. I knew I had to fight with all I had or I could give up. That's when I put everything I had into it. It's feeling that you have control over your life and what happens to you, even under the worse conditions.

Nancy — A friend of mine was in a coma for thirty-five days. The doctors told his parents that if he came out of it he'd be a vegetable, they'd have to put him in an institution. They were told he was never going to walk or talk again. And his parents said, "No, we'll take him home, we'll take care of him." Now he's going to school, he's talking and he drives. He was determined to show that the doctors were wrong by saying, "I'm going to beat this, I'm going to walk again and talk again."

Linda — I have a friend who was in the hospital and chose not to go through treatment. He said, "I want to go home." The doctors said, "You won't make it home." He was in bed for about a month at home and all of a sudden he started feeling that the will to live was what was going to keep him going. The last time I stopped by to see him, he didn't have time because he was going out to play tennis. He has leukemia and his white cells are extremely high, but his quality of life is also extremely high. Doctors need to be honest with their patients, yes, but not take away their hope. Don't tell them that they can't recover, because sometimes they can recover.

Nancy — And tell the patients that they have a choice. If you think there's no choice, you're not going to fight, you're not going to want to live.

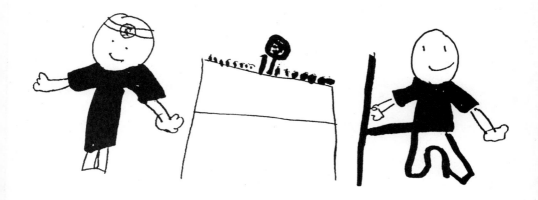

My sister Christina taught us all to live in the moment. You are not going to have it forever. Live all you can. She taught love, lots of love. She made me more aware of being sensitive about people's feelings and about how valuable life is.

—Jessica St. Germaine

Chapter 10

What It's Like for the Family

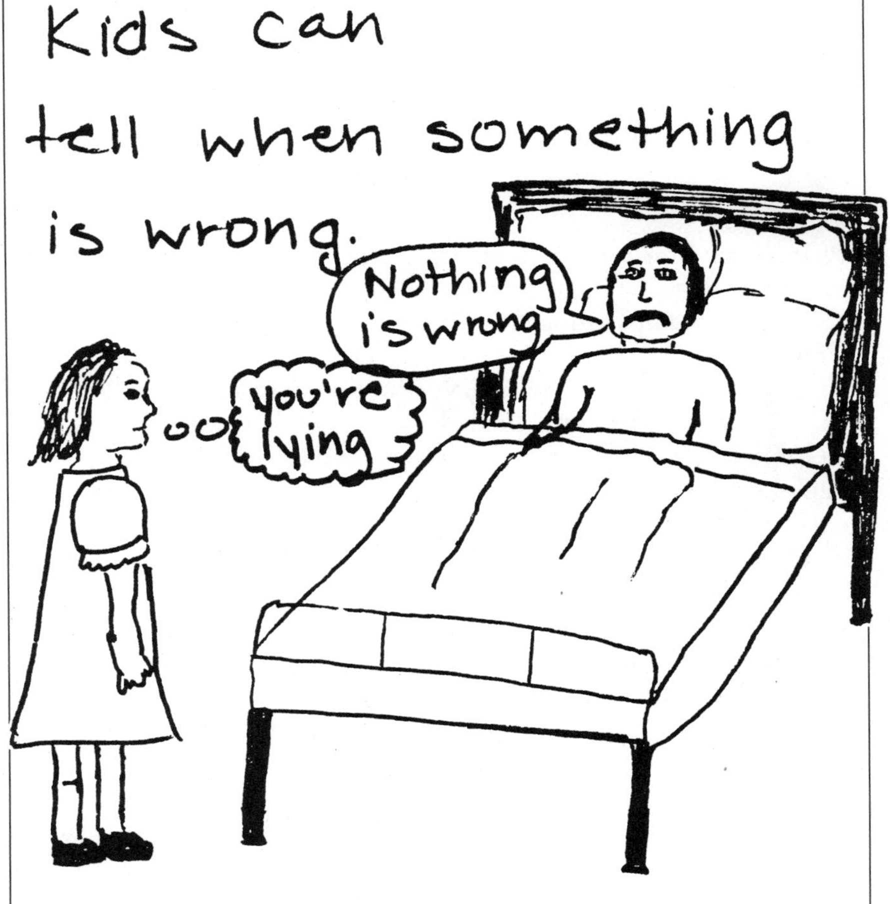

We're not the only ones going through our illness — our mothers and fathers, our brothers and sisters, are experiencing it with us. Sometimes it's a parent who's sick, and as sons and daughters we have our own set of insights and concerns.

Having gone through my mom's illness, I definitely feel differently now about myself. Not for everybody but I think for a lot of people, they're suddenly on a different level. I wouldn't say a higher level, but a different level of looking at the world, a different view somehow.

—*Maria Immel*

It's important for parents to recognize that they have choices. Our son had such a hard time with CAT scans. It got so bad that they'd end up calling an anesthesiologist to put him out completely just to have a CAT scan, when the CAT scan itself is painless. So we arranged to have him taken on a field trip to the radiology department. He had a name tag that said he was a doctor and he was in charge. He got to push the buttons on the machine while all the technicians got on the table. They worked a lot with him on feeling in control. When he had his next CAT scan, he cried a little bit, but when he was done he got up on the table and gave the thumbs up sign. Now, when he has a CAT scan scheduled, we take him in a couple of days early to meet the technicians who will be on that day, so he'll know them by name.

—*Anne and Marc Elias*

While visiting family back east, I took my son to a new children's cancer clinic there. He was overwhelmed when he first walked in. The main lobby was spacious and well-lit, with aquariums helping to provide a peaceful atmosphere. The waiting room for the children was enormous. It had video machines (no quarters needed) and a stereo, games from Candyland to Monopoly, puzzles and art projects, a basketball hoop and nerf ball, plus tables, comfy chairs and big rocking chairs for the parents. There were staff members doing art projects and playing with the children. It was wonderful to see that the clinic and doctors, as well as the community, know how important it is to make the experience of childhood cancer as positive as it can be. I hope someday there will be clinics like this everywhere.

—Tricia Ward

I would definitely have family meetings available free of charge. While it takes up time and time is money, I don't think that doctors are that short of cash to have to charge for meetings. Not charging any more than you need to is a very good idea because I think a lot of people feel they're being cheated by doctors.

—Maria Immel

I don't think a soul in that whole hospital should be treated for cancer, have chemotherapy or even surgery, unless they are also set up with a family counselor.

——Shirley Fraser

The first time the doctor told me my mother only had six months to live, it really upset me. Then she lived two years after they said that, so I began not to trust the doctor.
It was only after I'd had a long relationship with this doctor, because my mother had been sick for so long, that it got to the point where the doctor would tell me what was happening. And it was also at the point where it was really serious, when my mother was very ill. Up until then, no doctor told me anything. My mother's radiation doctors showed my brother and me the whole layout, where people lay and where the treatment was, the machines and all, and I really liked that because people finally explained what was going on.

—*Maria Immel*

I would not have such strict visiting hours, unless the child could not handle it. They need to be with their families as much as possible.

—*Jessica St. Germaine*

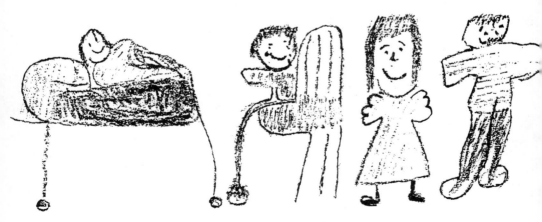

If a show that our son wanted to watch was on television and a nurse had to give him a shot, she would wait until his show was over. There was only one nurse that I didn't like. I asked her for an aspirin because my head was splitting and she just said, "I could get sued for that."

—*Tricia Ward*

One of the nurses gave us Bernie Siegel's *Love, Medicine and Miracles* and we asked the oncologist if she'd read this book. She said no, she didn't have time. In my opinion most oncology doctors act as if it would be so much easier if the disease were in a test tube where they could work on it, not in a human being. In a test tube they wouldn't have to talk to it.

—*Shirley Fraser*

I thought a lot about my mother having cancer, but I thought if I didn't say anything, maybe it would help my dad not feel the pain so much. I think basically I tucked it inside and tried to work it out inside myself. It didn't seem like asking medical questions was going to make any difference—that wasn't what it was about.

—*Maria Immel*

I asked my daughter if she wanted to get some emotional support through the hospital, because there are counselors there who would talk to her, and she said, "Mom, there are only about three days out of every three weeks that I feel good, and the last thing I want to do on one of those days is talk to some doctor about how bad I feel!"

—*Shirley Fraser*

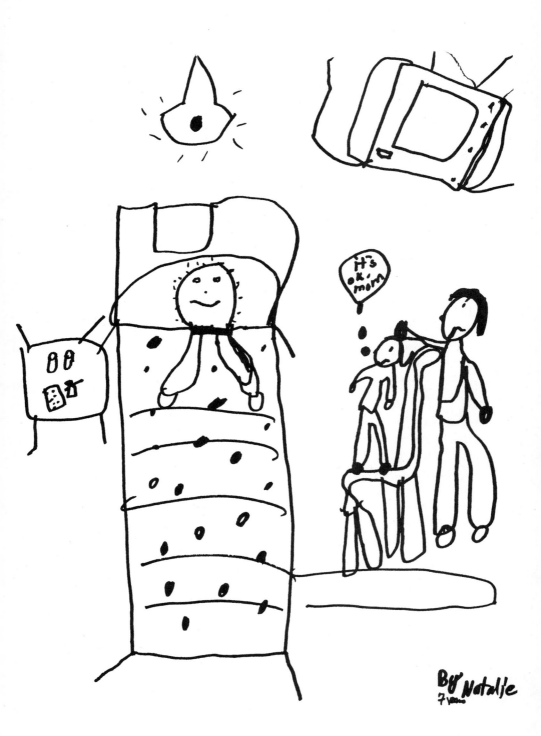

Her brother always treated her like a sister, not like a sick person. He helped keep normalcy in her life by treating her as one of the family, not like a little china doll.

—*Pam Marconi*

We are basically a loud family, all of us. But we quieted down a lot for her sake, because she was easily excited and when she was excited, it made it difficult for her to breathe. We tried to share moments with her. I believe that it's pulled us together a lot more. She taught us how to be strong.

—*Jessica St. Germaine*

For the situation being what it was, it couldn't have been much better. There was a bed in the room for us, so we could stay with our son. The doctors were really good, they cared, they were supportive, they wanted our son to know what was going on, they really involved the parents. When they had things to tell us, they would let our son decide if he wanted them to tell us in front of him or outside his room. If he didn't want them to come in, they didn't come in. They really listened to the children.

—*Tricia and Michael Ward*

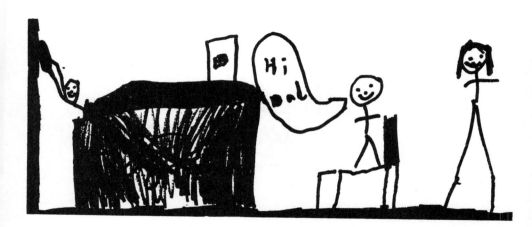

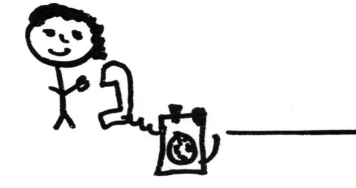

Advice to Kids

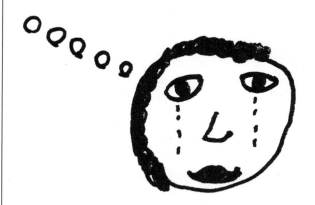

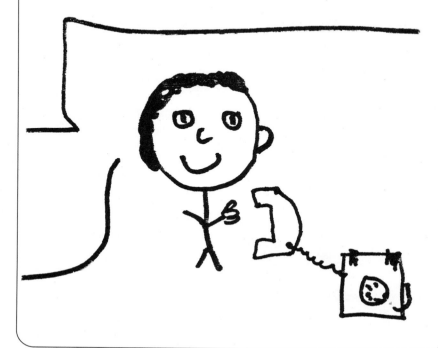

Think positively. Otherwise, you'll make it harder than it has to be. Your mental attitude has a lot to do with it.

—*Ricky Alaniz*

Shut your eyes and pretend that your mother is there. Think about your favorite place. Talk to the nurses. They'll say everything will be alright. They will probably help a little — more than the doctors. Doctors will scare you pretty much. They probably won't talk to you at all. Don't worry.

—*Rhonda Bruntmeyer*

When you go into the hospital, just understand that the things that are going to happen are to help you rather than just to make you feel bad. Once you understand what you're going in for, it'll help you deal with what you're going through.

—*Kenny Estrada*

For me, the worst thing was my thinking that it was never going to be better. I think it's been really important for me and my coping with my illness, just to try to live today, try to live in the moment and not think about the future.

—*Eve Nadel*

This is what I tried to think of to get well.

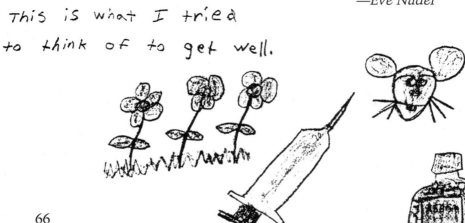

Try not to be scared. Squeeze the truth out of the doctors. When they say it's not going to hurt, tell them, "Bull fudge." Expect the worst, but try for the best. Try and think good thoughts, because it won't always be that bad, it just seems that way. Be open with your doctors, nurses and family because it doesn't help to keep things locked up inside. When you're feeling down, let your feelings out, because they'll eventually blow up and take you for an uncomfortable ride. Last but not least, *always* look on the bright side of life because it's one thing you always have going for you, as long as you choose to look that way.

—*Noah Wolfson*

I found a way around the food. I was talking with one of the nurses, saying, "Everything that they have on here, I hate." She said, "Well, there's something you can do. If there's nothing on there that you want, just write down hamburger. They'll always give you that." One time, I jokingly asked for pizza. I got my menu sent back to me saying, "Ha ha ha, we ain't buying you no pizza!" So I just said, "Hey, send me down a hamburger."

—*Justin Gregoire*

One of the things I liked a lot was that I had so many visitors.

—*Peter Elias*

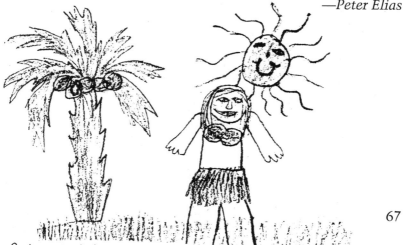

Robert Griffith age 10

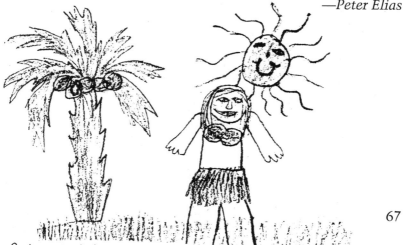

When I was in the hospital, my Snoopy helped me. It was something personal for me to hold. Maybe having a picture of a member of your family, things like a familiar blanket from home or a pillow, something that you're used to, would be nice. When something was fearful, I thought about it and examined it and tried to figure things out. It helped me to have information. If you're blocking it out and it's still pushing its way in, I think the best way is just to look at it. Listening to music somehow relaxes me and makes it possible for me to look at what I'm doing and examine myself without getting into the emotional stuff, crying and yelling and screaming that I would have done earlier.

—*Maria Immel*

You can't let the treatment worry you and interfere with the rest of your life. If it bogs you down, it will make you depressed or mad. Doctors should always listen to everything you say. Otherwise they're not good doctors. But you have to prepare what you're going to say to them so they know everything that's going on.

—*John Crandall*

This is what
I'm going to d
when I get well

68

Just kind of tell them what you want. And you have to be confident, you have to say, "I can get through this and I'm not going to die." If you just give up and say, "Well, whatever's gonna happen is whatever's gonna happen," or "This is too hard," or "I can't do it," you're not going to make it. But if you say you can do it, you can.

—*Sarah Cox*

My advice to patients: Don't worry, because the divine plan is with you always and trust that.

—*Kelly Niles*

To me, doctors are people that maybe you can trust, who know about what's going on with you inside your body and who are willing to explain it to you. I've always found it easy to talk to doctors. Once you learn about the thing and how to deal with it, you feel better about yourself and you can talk better with the doctors, too. But it's up to you to make the first move.

—*Kenny Estrada*

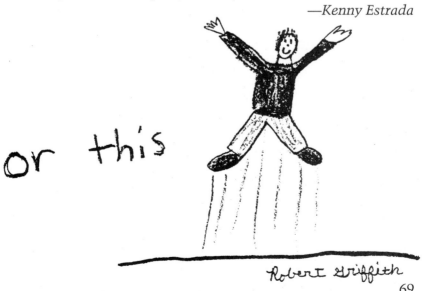

or this

Robert Griffith

I kind of look at myself before I was sick and I just can't believe I'm the same person. I've changed so much. In a way, I like myself better.

—Sarah Cox

Chapter 12

Who We Are

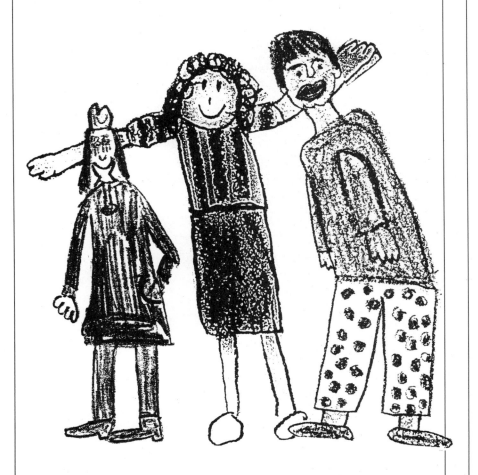

Frankie

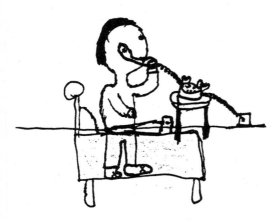

The kids (and their families) who wrote and illustrated this book all came to the Center for Attitudinal Healing during their illness. Their contributions to the book were part of an ongoing project for several years. While putting the book together in the fall of 1990, the editors spoke again with as many of the families as we could contact to learn how their lives were progressing.

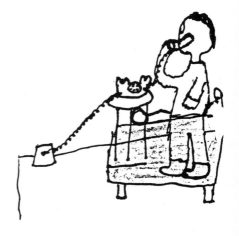

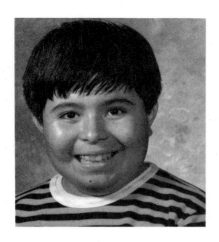

Ricky Alaniz had a bout of pneumonia when he was five that left him with weak lungs; otherwise, he had a normal childhood. He loved to build model cars and airplanes. Just after his thirteenth birthday, he complained of headaches and nausea and was diagnosed with a brain tumor. Radiation and chemotherapy treatment removed the tumor and Ricky was able to finish eighth grade. The chemo had side effects, however, that impacted his lungs. Too weak to begin high school, he spent the rest of his life at home with his family, studying his special interest, astronomy. He was eventually confined to a wheelchair, breathing with the help of an oxygen unit. Ricky died of lung failure at the age of seventeen.

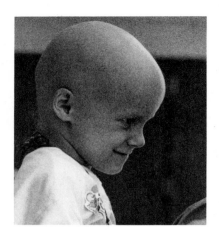

Melissa Callen had just turned four when she was diagnosed with rhabdomyo-sarcoma. This uncommon tumor developed in her nasal sinuses and was obstructing her ability to breathe. Because her symptoms were similar to those of a sinus infection, it took six weeks for her illness to be diagnosed. She received radiation treatment, which made her very ill, and she was on chemotherapy for almost two and a half years. She went into remission when she was six, and her checkups have found no evidence of recurrence. While Melissa was in treatment, she couldn't be around other children because of her fragile immune system. Now she is thrilled to be able to go to school with her friends.

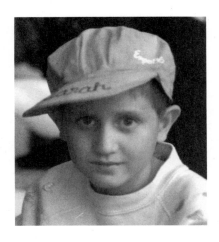

Sarah Cox was diagnosed with leukemia when she was seven. Radiation and chemotherapy treatment brought the cancer into remission, with monthly chemo follow-ups. Despite missing half of second grade, she is an A student. Sarah says of her experience with cancer, "I kind of look at myself before I was sick and I just can't believe I'm the same person. I've changed so much. In a way, I like myself better."

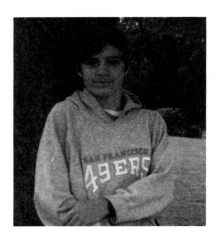

John Crandall was surfing at Stinson Beach with some of his eighth grade buddies after school, when he became very nauseated and got a sudden, almost unbearable, headache. The staff of a neighborhood diner were able to quiet his screaming, crying and vomiting until an ambulance arrived. Six hours later, he was diagnosed with a slow-growing but now hemor-rhaging brain tumor, and nine hours of surgery followed. The prognosis was not encouraging; his doctors thought the tumor would promptly recur. John, how-ever, had no doubt from the beginning that he would recover. When radiation was administered for six weeks and the tumor did not grow, his doctors became cautiously optimistic. Chemotherapy

followed for another year and a half. John so wanted to graduate with his eighth grade class that his teacher provided special tutoring for him. At the graduation, he played his own piano arrangement of "The Star Spangled Banner." In high school, he had the full support of the school staff to care for his health first. He grew spiritually during this time and that trust in spirit became his support toward health. John is now at Brigham Young University, where he is an avid student of music, foreign languages and religion.

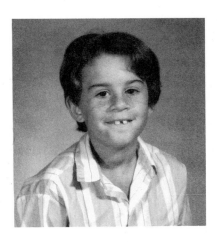

Peter Elias complained of
terrible headaches when he
was almost six; X-rays showed
a dark shadow and the CAT
scan pictured a massive brain
tumor. His was diagnosed a
slow-growing tumor, with a
two-to-ten-year life expec-
tancy. Peter has had no
response to radiation treatments. While tests show no
growth in the tumor, his
condition is not clear: the
tumor may yet be growing,
it may be dormant, or it may
have become fibrotic (a benign
mass of scar tissue). Today
Peter is enjoying every
moment.

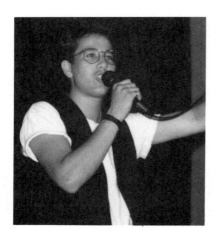

Kenny Estrada was one of the children who founded the Center for Attitudinal Healing, when he was a five-year-old with leukemia. He spent the first year of his chemotherapy treatment in the hospital, then continued to be treated intermittently until the age of twelve. He wrote his "advice to doctors" about that time. Kenny has continued to be in good health since he went into remission. Now grown up, he manages a store and plans to go to college for a business degree. He was one of the authors of the Center's first book by children, *There Is A Rainbow Behind Every Dark Cloud.*

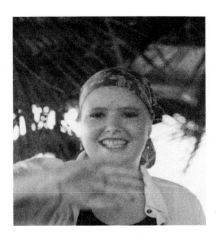

Valerie Fraser's severe back pain, when she was sixteen, was attributed by her pediatrician to a fall in the shower. When she continued in such intense pain that she was unable to sleep, her chiropractor suggested she be checked "to see if she was well in other ways." An X-ray showed a large tumor on her backbone. In the next three years, Valerie had three operations, radiation, and chemotherapy; however, the tumor continued to grow. When it became clear that they were unable to arrest the tumor, Valerie's doctors suggested she make the most of the time she had. She went to the Caribbean, then spent Thanksgiving and Christmas with her family, under hospice care. Valerie died at home at age nineteen, with the insight, her mother states, of a thirty-year-old.

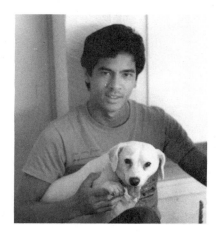

Earl Garcia's parents gave him body-building equipment for his sixteenth birthday, because he wanted to bulk up for varsity sports. When he began to complain of muscle pains, they were dismissed as growing pains. Then, during a family ski trip, he began to stumble and lose his balance. A CAT scan found a tumor putting pressure on the spine, which was operated on immediately. While the bulk of the tumor was removed, fear of nerve damage and paralysis had stopped the surgeons from getting it all. With follow-up chemotherapy, Earl spent the next four and a half years in remission, being very physically and mentally active. He coached three Little League teams and he twice ran in San Francisco's Bay to Breakers race, finishing in the first 17,000 of 200,000 runners. He completed high school and went on to become an architectural drafting technician, graduating with honors. He worked for an architectural firm while continuing his studies. Then another tumor was found. After another round of chemo, Earl elicited a promise from his family that he would not have to go through chemo again or ever be put on life-support systems. During the more than a year that followed, outliving his doctors' expectations, Earl played tennis, water-skied, sailed, bicycled and jogged. His ability to be totally present, to choose peace and share love in every moment, was an inspiration to all who knew him. His friends considered him a warrior of the heart. Earl lived fully, then died from massive brain hemorrhaging at the age of twenty-two.

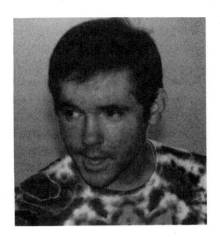

Justin Gregoire was sixteen
when he started to get bad
headaches and was diagnosed
with a brain tumor the size of
a golf ball. Most of the tumor
was removed in surgery and
more of it through follow-up
radiation at Harvard, using
heavy proton-beam radiation.
He still has the tumor today
and it is getting smaller and
smaller. When he was twenty-
four, he had surgery to
completely remove an off-
shoot of the original tumor.
Justin is on medication to
prevent seizures. He's feeling
fantastic and maintaining his
wonderful sense of humor.

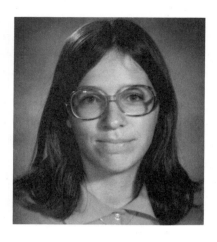

Maria Immel was about five when her mother developed melanoma. Her mom underwent treatment and went into remission. The cancer reappeared, however, and she died when Maria was ten. A year later, Maria's father was hospitalized with kidney cancer. Maria herself has spent eleven days in the hospital recovering from an emergency appendectomy. She is now in high school — a serious student and an accomplished violist.

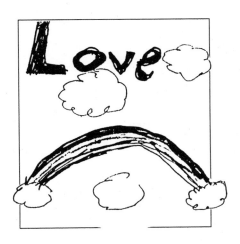

Christina Marconi was
eighteen months-old when she
contracted AIDS through a
blood transfusion. She
developed chronic lung
disease, requiring continuous
oxygen therapy. She was
hospitalized then, again a year
later, and a third time at age
five. Though most of her short
life was spent with constant
medical care, Christina
touched everyone she met
with her energy, innocent
insight and wisdom. Her life's
dream of visiting Disneyland
was fulfilled; she spoke with
Mary Poppins and sailed the
skies with Dumbo. She died at
home, surrounded by her
family, at the age of six.

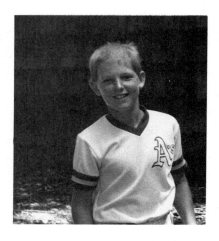

Liam McCauley was just past three when he started bleeding from his nose and mouth. The diagnosis was acute lymphocytic leukemia. He completed a year of chemotherapy and was completely well until he relapsed just before his eighth birthday. He then received three more years of treatment, and has been healthy since then. He wrote about his experience for this book when he was eleven and completing treatment. For a time, Liam was small for his age, but, at age sixteen, he stood six feet tall. He seldom speaks about the leukemia, preferring to move forward with his life.

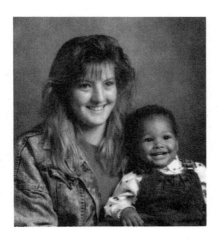

Margaret McDonald was born with a Wilm's kidney tumor, which in most children appears by age five. Hers, however, remained dormant until she had symptoms that resembled appendicitis when she was twelve. After a year of medical complications, including an appendectomy and surgery for a twisted bowel, the Wilm's tumor was finally discovered, a kidney removed and chemotherapy begun. Her regular checkups continue to be encouraging. In the meantime, Margaret has become a busy young mother and college student. At fifteen, she delivered a beautiful baby boy, Sean. At sixteen, she passed the high school proficiency test and at seventeen, she enrolled at the College of Marin. Margaret plans to teach kindergarten.

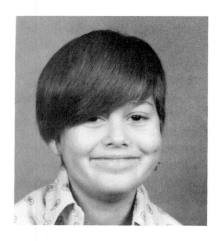

Quincy Munch was born with congenital heart disease. When he was five years-old, his heart failed and he had a valve replaced. He had a tracheostomy when he was seven and another heart valve replaced when he was nine. At age thirteen, Quincy was one of the youngest people ever to receive a heart transplant. This photograph was taken on Quincy's first day back at school after recuperating from his transplant surgery. At eighteen, he's on medication and his activities are not restricted.

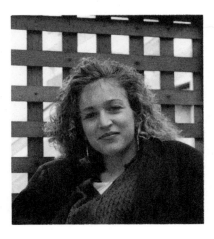

Eve Nadel developed chronic pain, anorexia and depression when she was sixteen. She was in so much pain her last year of high school that she missed three months of school and didn't go to her graduation. At age eighteen, she joined the Young Adults Group at the Center for Attitudinal Healing. She has been hospitalized, had vascular surgery and been on pain, antidepressant and gastric medications, none of which worked for her. However, Eve has now overcome her anorexia. She sees the Center, where she is a member of the Board and in training to be a group facilitator, as a place of safety where she can grow and heal herself. She has worked as a hospital lab assistant and as a psychiatric nurse assistant.

She is a full-time student at San Francisco State University, studying philosophy, writing and film.

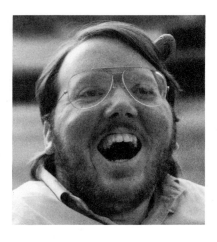

Kelly Niles was eleven and playing baseball when he fought with a bigger boy over who had the next turn at bat. He was punched several times in the head. His dad took him to the emergency room, where he had an X-ray that was incorrectly read. He was sent home. Within hours, with severe symptoms, they returned to the emergency room; a more experienced doctor noted epidural hematoma and scheduled surgery. Despite two surgeries and intense physical therapy, Kelly lapsed into a six-week coma. He spent a year and a half in the hospital, tube fed, with no muscular control. The doctors believed that Kelly's mental capacity had been affected and recommended that he be permanently institutionalized. His parents felt, however, that Kelly was alert, and his mom took him home and cared for him herself. Eventually, Kelly could sit in a wheelchair with a tray and use his arm to move toward one side of the tray for yes, the other side for no. With the financial settlements from malpractice suits, Kelly now has twenty-four hour attendant care and can communicate, with a special computer, the extraordinary thoughts of his very active mind. He loves music and has extensively studied philosophy, psychology and spirituality. Kelly, at 30, has been learning to find inner peace and shares that peace and love with everyone he encounters. He trusts that everything has a purpose, and says, "I take this viewpoint because it works."

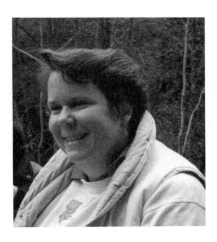

Nancy Peugh was the only girl of the original kids who started the Center. An active eleven year-old, busy keeping pace with her five sisters and brothers, she began to have side aches when running. After numerous evaluations, a tumor on her kidney was discovered; the kidney was removed. She had chemo and radiation therapy every day for the next two years. From the middle of fifth grade to the beginning of eighth, she studied via a home tutor. Life returned to normal. Then, ten years later, early signs of cervical cancer showed up. Nancy drove herself to the hospital for the outpatient operation, and drove herself home the same day. She is currently an instructional aide working with school children who have special educational needs.

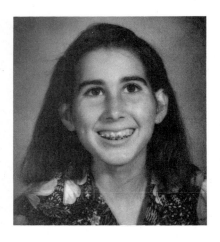

Marina Rozen began, around
her third birthday, to show
subtle symptoms that developed into staggering and a loss
of coordination. She told her
parents it felt like "kids are
hitting me." Her pediatrician
suspected a brain tumor and
called in a neurosurgeon who,
after further study, scheduled
surgery. Although the tumor
was successfully removed,
other complications developed
that resulted in severe
learning disabilities as well as
other problems. At 16, she
attends special day classes in
a public school.

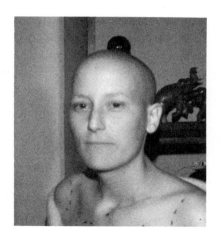 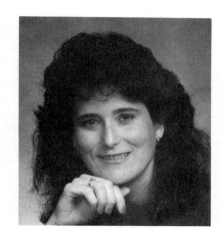

Linda Stover, a real people-person, enjoyed a large circle of friends as she grew toward adulthood. She loved to write poetry in her quieter moments, too. Just before her twenty-first birthday, she began having problems with breathing and thought she had asthma. Non-Hodgkins lymphoma was diagnosed, however. She attributes her success in fighting the cancer through ten long months of chemotherapy to her faith and strong will to live. Now, with all that long behind her, she works for the radiation oncologist who treated her and volunteers in the Young Adults Group at the Center—giving as she once received.

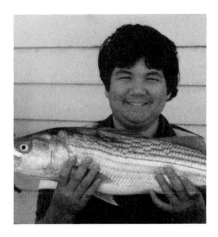

Bobby Toops learned to sign before he learned to speak, because his parents are both deaf. He enjoys a close relationship with his parents and his sister Tina and he likes to go fishing with his dad. When he was eight, his mom first noticed blood in his urine. He was diagnosed with glomerulonephritis, an inflammation of the kidneys. Three years later he had a kidney transplant, using a kidney donated by his father. Bobby signed his doctors' comments to his parents when interpreters were not available, even from his hospital bed. The disease returned after five years, so he underwent a second transplant when he was sixteen. Today his medication is closely monitored and he receives thorough check-ups every two months. However, he lives life fully. Currently he is in college studying electical engineering and computers, is filling a wall with trophies won from assembling and racing radio-controlled model cars, and entertains friends with juggling acts.

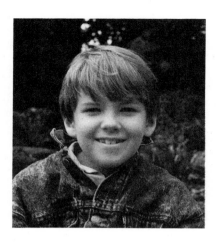

Zack Ward was six years old
when a lump was found on his
neck; his parents thought he'd
been bitten by a tick. He was
given antibiotics. When his
fever shot up, tests were done
and his doctors diagnosed a
high-risk T-cell acute
lymphocytic leukemia. Zack
immediately started two
months of intense radiation
on Halloween, wearing his
vampire costume to the
hospital. His three year
chemotherapy program
finished on New Year's
Day. What a way to begin
the new year!

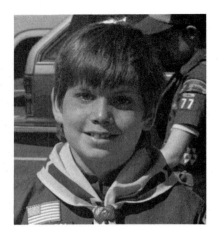

Andrew Watt collected stamps and coins as a young boy. About age eight he began to have violent headaches, nausea, dizziness and double vision. Doctors at first were unable to diagnose his problem, but quickly treated his acute hydrocephalus. They eventually discovered a tumor of the brain, but offered little hope for recovery. After a long three month search, an experienced and caring physician was found to treat Andrew. A fourteen-hour biopsy was performed, and, two weeks later, a sixteen-hour operation. The radiation therapy that followed for a hundred days was relatively painless. Andrew had some problems after the treatment—eyes crossed, double vision, and a staggering gait. These problems turned out to be temporary, however. After three years with no sign of recurrence, Andrew lives the life of a normal twelve year-old, collecting baseball cards and noticing girls.

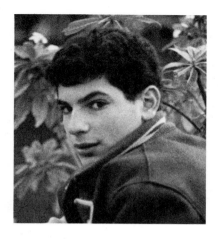

Noah Wolfson was diagnosed with acute lymphocytic leukemia when he was twelve. Extensive chemotherapy brought the disease into remission for eighteen months. Because of a bad drug reaction, however, his doctors stopped chemotherapy. Two relapses followed. Noah elected to have a bone marrow transplant in Seattle. He told his parents, "I want to take my chance. If there's only a one percent chance, I want to take it. Don't take my chance away." When the transplant did not take, he asked to go home for the last week of his life. Four days before he died, he spoke to an assembly at his high school. He said good-bye to his classmates, speaking with candor, love and bravery to them about his illness, his impending death, and their own precious lives. Two days later, he went for a last swim, shortly before going into a coma, then died at the age of sixteen.

Rhonda Bruntmeyer received radiation treatment for a rare cancerous tumor on her spine when she was five.

Josh Engholm was nine years old when he had cirrohsis of the liver and hyperspleenism; he also underwent an ileostomy.

These children participated in the Children's Group at the Center in the early 1980s. Since then the Center has lost contact with their families.

We wish them love wherever they are.

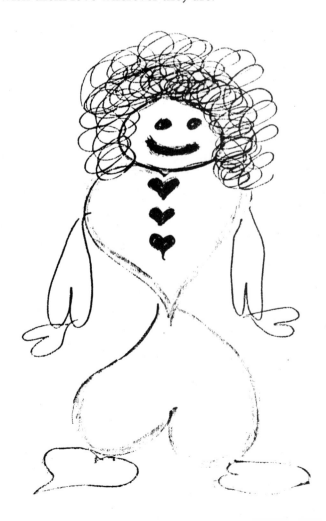

Further Reading
Books Written by Children on Living with Illness

"In Grade one when I was five years old I got pains in the belly and got sick. The doctor said I had to go to the hospital and have an operation because I had a lump in my belly."

Bannah, Joe. **My Treatment.** Queensland, Australia: Boolarong Publications, 1982. Available through The Children's Leukemia and Cancer Society, P.O. Box 361, North Brisbane, Queensland, 400, Australia. An account of two years of treatment for non-Hodgkins lymphoma, written by an Australian boy.

— ♥ —

Bergman, Thomas. **One Day at a Time: Children Living with Cancer.** Wake Forest, North Carolina: Stevens, 1989. This book includes interviews with kids.

— ♥ —

"My mother said, 'You're not going to die.'" "Did you believe her?" "Hey, when your mother says something you don't dare question it." — Ann, age 10.

Bombeck, Erma. **I Want to Grow Hair, I Want to Grow Up, I Want to Go to Boise: Children Surviving Cancer.** New York: Harper & Row, 1989. "... We meet kids and their families conquering the most difficult times of all. Along the way we get to know mothers, fathers, siblings, friends, schoolmates, relatives, doctors, and teachers."

— ♥ —

"This is a book written for children like us who have gotten sick with cancer, leukemia, and other sicknesses where you are scared you might die. We find as we help each other, we help ourselves. We hope that writing this small book will help you gain through sharing our experiences."

Center for Attitudinal Healing. **There is a Rainbow Behind Every Dark Cloud.** Berkeley, CA: Celestial Arts, 1978.

"I think this book had to be written for all kids who find out that their brother or sister is sick with a catastrophic illness. By reading about other people who have had the same thing happen to them, they will understand that they aren't the only people who have these problems, and they may discover how to handle these problems. When I first discovered my little brother had leukemia there was no book like this around to help me, and so I had to handle these problems myself." — Stephen Bird, age 13.

Center for Attitudinal Healing. **Another Look at the Rainbow.** Berkeley, CA: Celestial Arts, 1982.

— ♥ —

"The rezin I wanted to write a book about having cansur is because . . . I want to tell kids you dont always die. If you get cansur dont be scared cause lots of people get over having cansur and grow up without dying."

Gaes, Jason. **My Book for Kids with Cansur: A Child's Autobiography of Hope.** Aberdeen, South Dakota: Melius & Peterson. 1987. Written by an eight-year-old boy and illustrated by his brothers.

— ♥ —

Graelle, Karen & Bertram, John. **Teenagers Face-to-Face with Cancer.** Englewood Cliffs, New Jersey: Messner, 1986. The teenagers who helped write this book talk about their emotional and medical experiences with cancer.

"It's now been six years since I was diagnosed with cancer and . . . my attitude toward the cancer has changed over the years. I used to think it was a really terrible thing; now I know it's something that has really helped me as a person." — Julie C., age 18.

Kjosness, Mary A. & Rudolph, Laura., Editors. **What Happened to You Happened to Me.** American Cancer Society, 1984. Written and illustrated by children with cancer, ages 6 to 19, at The Children's Orthopedic Hospital and Medical Center in Seattle, Washington.

— ♥ —

"Sometimes I wonder if . . . anyone will want to marry me because my children may have diabetes . . . My mother told me that it wouldn't be a problem because when people are really in love, the relationship comes first. My brother says I shouldn't even be thinking about marriage for another fifteen years. He's right! Besides, by then there may be a cure for diabetes. In the meantime, things are okay because no matter what happens, I'm still me." — Rachel Demaster, age 10.

Krementz, Jill. **How It Feels To Fight For Your Life.** Boston: Little, Brown, 1989. Fourteen children, from 7 to 16, dealing with serious illnesses and disabilities, share "their fears, their hopes, and their sources of strength and support."

— ♥ —

"I know that you will be able to handle cancer. Becaus if I can you can. It's o.k. to be scard. You hav to hav a positiv aditud. Say to yourself you can do anything. Never say you can't. You just hav to hang in ther! I think you can do it. I rote this book to help people with cancer. Your not alone."

Lancaster, Mathew. **Hang Toughf.** New York: Paulist Press, 1985.

"One day [my friend] asked me whether the tumor was malignant or benign . . . whether I would get better and what would happen to me — and I could tell by his questions and the way he asked, that he really cared about me. That was the beginning of my fight for life."

Porter, Garrett & Norris, Patricia A., Phd., **Why Me? Harnessing the Healing Power of the Human Spirit.** Walpole, New Hampshire: Stillpoint Publishing, 1985. Written by a nine-year-old boy and his therapist about their partnership, using visualization and imagery, as a successful approach to his cancer treatment.